CROCKPOT

50 Delicious Slow Cooker Recipes For Healthy Living And Weight Loss -- Crockpot Recipes Books (Paleo Slow Cooker, Instant Pot Cookbook and Recipes, Electric Pressure Cooker)

By CINDY FLAVORS

Table of Contents

Copyright Notice

Disclaimer

Chapter One – Healthy Living Crockpot Breakfast Recipes

Apple Granola Crumble

Ingredients

- 2 Apples
- 1 C. Granola Cereal
- ⅛ C. Maple Syrup
- ¼ C. Apple Juice
- 2 Tbsp. Vegan Butter
- 1 Tsp. Cinnamon
- ½ Tsp. Nutmeg

Directions

1. Peel and core the apples. Then cut them into thick slices and then into chunks. You can accomplish this by cutting the apple in half and then halve those halves. This will give you eight thick slices. Cut those slices into chunks, around three per slice.
2. Add everything to your slow cooker and stir.
3. Cover and cook on low for four hours.

Slow Cooker, Banana & Coconut Milk Steel-Cut Oatmeal

Ingredients

- 2 Bananas, Sliced
- 28 Oz. Canned Light Coconut Milk
- ½ C. Water
- 1 C. Steel Cut Oats
- 2 Tbsp. Brown Sugar
- 1-½ Tbsp. Butter
- ½ Tsp. Cinnamon
- ¼ Tsp. Nutmeg
- ½ Tsp. Vanilla
- 1 Tbsp. Ground Flax Seed
- ¼ Tsp. Salt

Directions

1. Coat the inside of your slow cooker with some cooking spray. Add everything to the slow cooker. Stir and cook on low for seven hours, covered. Spoon it into bowls and add some toppings. Store the leftovers in the refrigerator. You can also store it in the freezer.

2. To reheat it, put a single serving in the microwave and add a third of a cup of milk. Microwave on high for one minute, stir and then microwave another minute or until it's hot.

Carrot Cake Zucchini Bread Oatmeal

Ingredients

- ½ C. Steel-Cut Oats
- 1½ C. Vanilla-Flavored Non-Dairy Milk
- 1 Small Carrot, Grated
- ¼ Small Zucchini, Peeled And Grated
- Pinch Of Nutmeg
- Pinch Of Salt
- Pinch Of Ground Cloves
- ½ Tsp. Cinnamon
- 2 Tbsp. Brown Sugar
- ¼ C. Chopped Pecans
- 1 Tsp. Of Pure Vanilla Extract

Directions

1. The night before, oil the slow cooker and combine all the ingredients, but the pecans, in the slow cooker. Cook on low for eight hours.
2. Stir it, taste, and adjust your seasonings. Add more milk if you need to. Top it with the pecans.

Coconut Cranberry Crockpot Quinoa

Ingredients

- 3 C. Coconut Water
- 1 C. Quinoa, Uncooked

- 1 Tsp. Vanilla Extract
- 3 Tsp. Honey
- ½ C. Coconut Flakes
- ½ C. Almonds, Sliced
- ¼ C. Cranberries, Dried

1. Put everything into a slow cooker and cook on low for four hours or on high for two hours. This makes about three cups cooked.

Creamy Homemade Yogurt

- 3 Tsp. Grass-Fed Gelatin
- ½ Gallon Organic Milk
- 6 Oz. Plain Organic Yogurt With Live Cultures
- ½ C. Pure Maple Syrup
- 1 ½ Tbsp. Pure Vanilla Extract

1. Pour half a gallon of milk into the slow cooker and cook for three hours on low or until the mixture reaches a temperature between 150 and 175 degrees Fahrenheit.

2. Ladle out half to one cup of the milk into a bowl and add the gelatin a teaspoon at a time, whisking. Return the mix back to the slow cooker and give it all a good whisk. If you mix it gradually, there should be no lumps, but if you do see some, use a fine mesh

strainer to pour the mix back into the slow cooker to remove any lumps.

3. Turn off your slow cooker and let the milk rest two to three hours or until the mix has cooled to around 110 degrees Fahrenheit. If it's 115 degrees or above, the bacteria will begin to be damaged.

4. Ladle half a cup of milk from the slow cooker and into a bowl. Whisk in the starter and add this mix back to the slow cooker. Give it a few gentle stirs and then cover it with a few large towels or a large blanket and let it incubate for eight to twelve hours. The slow cooker should be off during this step! The longer the incubation, the higher the acidity will be in the yogurt and the tarter it will be.

5. If the ambient temperature in your home is below 70 degrees Fahrenheit, it's hard for the cultures to work. If your home is cooler than 70 degrees, then consider putting a heat lamp nearby.

6. Remove around six ounces of plain yogurt and reserve it as a starter for the following batch. Add the ingredients for the vanilla flavoring. The yogurt will keep firming up once it's refrigerated and keeps for a few weeks.

Greek Eggs Crockpot Breakfast Casserole

Ingredients

- 12 Eggs, Whisked
- ½ C. Milk
- 1 Tsp. Black Pepper
- ½ Tsp. Salt

- 1 Tbsp. Onion
- 1 Tsp. Garlic
- ½ C. Sun Dried Tomatoes
- 1 C. Baby Bella Mushrooms, Sliced
- 2 C. Spinach
- ½ C. Feta Cheese

Directions

1. Whisk the eggs with the pepper, salt, and the milk in a mixing bowl.
2. Add the red onion and the garlic.
3. Add the mushrooms, tomatoes, and the spinach.
4. Pour the mix into the slow cooker and set it to low, and then top with the cheese.
5. Slow cook on low for four to six hours.

Slow-Cooker Huevos Rancheros

Ingredients

- Nonstick Spray
- 10 Eggs
- 1 C. Half-And-Half
- 12 Oz. Shredded Monterey Jack
- ½ Tsp. Black Pepper
- ½ Tsp. Ancho Chili Powder
- 1 Garlic Clove, Minced
- 1 (4-Oz.) Can Chopped Green Chilies, Drained

- 10 Oz. Taco Sauce
- 8 Corn Tortillas
- Scallions, Avocado, Cilantro And Lime, For Garnish

Directions

1. Spray the inside of your slow cooker with some nonstick spray.
2. In a bowl, beat the eggs with the half and half and eight ounces of the cheese. Add the pepper and the chili powder and give it another good whisk. Stir in the chilies and garlic. Pour it into the slow cooker and cook on low for two hours, covered. Check it to be sure the edges are not burning.
3. Remove the lid and pour into the taco sauce, using the back of a spoon to cover the eggs with it evenly. Scatter the rest of the cheese all over and put the lid back on. Keep cooking on low for fifteen more minutes.
4. Allow it to cool a bit and then cut it into wedges and serve it with the warmed tortillas. Garnish it with some scallions and avocado, a little fresh lime juice, and some cilantro.

Slow Cooker Overnight Quinoa and Oats

Ingredients

- 1 ½ C. Steel Cut Oats
- ½ C. Quinoa
- 4 ½ C. Water, Or Almond Milk
- 4 Tbsp. Brown Sugar
- 2 Tbsp. Real Maple Syrup

- ¼ Tsp. Salt
- 1 ½ Tsp. Vanilla Extract
- ¼ Tsp. Cinnamon
- Milk
- Berries
- Sugar

Directions

1. Spray the slow cooker with some non-stick cooking spray. Don't skip this step.
2. In a strainer, rinse out the quinoa very well.
3. Combine the oats, quinoa, almond milk or water, brown sugar, syrup, vanilla, salt, and cinnamon in the slow cooker.
4. Stir it well and then set the slow cooker on low for six to seven hours or overnight. If it goes more than eight, it will become mushy.
5. Once you get up, turn off the heat immediately and transfer the quinoa to another bowl to stop the cooking process.
6. Serve with a bit of milk, berries, and some brown sugar, if you like.

Slow Cooker Frittata with Artichoke Hearts, Roasted Red Pepper, and Feta

Ingredients

- 1 14 Oz. Can Small Artichoke Hearts, Drained And Diced
- 1 12 Oz. Jar Roasted Red Peppers, Drained And Diced

- ¼ C. Green Onions, Sliced
- 8 Eggs, Beaten
- 4 Oz. Feta Cheese, Crumbled
- Black Pepper
- 2 Tbsp. Chopped Parsley

Directions

1. Pour the artichoke into a colander and put them in the sink so that they can drain well. While they drain, slice the onions and crumble the cheese. Spray the slow cooker with some non-stick cooking spray. Coat it well.

2. Remove the artichoke to the cutting board and pour out the roasted red peppers into the colander and let them drain. Dice the artichoke hearts into small pieces and put them in the bottom of your slow cooker. Cut the drained peppers into pieces about half an inch square and put them in the slow cooker. Add the sliced green onions to the slow cooker.

3. Beat the eggs until the yolks and whites are totally combined and pour the eggs over the vegetables in your slow cooker. Use a fork to stir it around gently, so that the red pepper, artichoke, and green onions are distributed throughout the eggs. Sprinkle with the cheese and season to taste with some pepper.

4. Cook on low two to three hours or until the eggs are firm and the cheese has melted.

5. Cut it into pieces while it's still in the slow cooker. Serve hot and sprinkle with some chopped parsley to garnish, if you'd like.

Slow Cooker Vegetable Omelet

Ingredients

- 6 Eggs
- ½ C. Milk
- ¼ Tsp. Salt
- Pepper
- ⅛ Tsp. Chili Powder
- ⅛ Tsp. Garlic Powder
- 1 C. Broccoli Florets
- 1 Small Yellow Onion, Finely Chopped
- 1 Red Bell Pepper, Thinly Sliced
- 1 Garlic Clove, Minced
- Chopped Tomatoes
- Shredded Cheddar Cheese
- Fresh Parsley
- Chopped Onions

Directions

1. Lightly grease your slow cooker insert with some cooking spray and set it aside.
2. In a mixing bowl, combine the milk, eggs, salt, garlic powder, pepper, and chili powder using an egg beater or a whisk. Beat the mix until it's well combined.
3. Add the sliced peppers, broccoli, garlic, and onions to the slow cooker and stir in the egg mix.

4. Cover and cook on high two hours. Begin checking for doneness after an hour and a half. The omelet is finished when the eggs are set.

5. Sprinkle it with cheese and let it rest two to three minutes or until the cheese is fully melted.

6. Turn off your slow cooker and cut the omelet into eight pieces.

7. Transfer it to a serving plate.

8. Garnish with the chopped onions, tomatoes, and the parsley.

9. Serve.

Chapter Two – Paleo Slow Cooker Lunch Recipes

Slow Cooker Puerco Pibil

Ingredients

- 15 Oz. Fire-Roasted Diced Tomato
- 1 Medium Onion
- 2 Tbsp. Annatto Powder
- 1 Tsp. Ground Cumin
- 1 Tsp. Salt
- 1 Tsp. Ground Black Pepper
- Pinch Of Nutmeg
- 5 Lbs. Pork Shoulder Roast
- 1 Orange, Juiced
- ¼ C. Apple Cider Vinegar
- 2 Tsp. Salt

Directions

1. In a bowl, mix the annatto, pepper, cumin, a teaspoon of salt, and a pinch of nutmeg together. Stir in a little water until it's like a thick, pasty consistency.

2. Slice the onion and add it to a skillet with a spoonful of fat, such as coconut oil or butter, over medium heat. Cook a few minutes until it's translucent, and then add the tomatoes. Cook another two to three minutes or until they're softened.

3. Prepare the pork by trimming off large pieces of external fat. If there's fat on the inside of the meat, most of it will cook out. Slice the roast into long pieces around an inch and a half wide. Season with some salt.

4. In the slow cooker, mix the juice of the orange with the vinegar. Add the spice paste and stir until it's dissolved. Put the pork into the liquid and top with the onion and tomato mix.

5. Cook on low six to eight hour. Skim off any excess fat while it's warm and refrigerate it so the rest of the fat is solidified. Scrape off the rest of the fat and store in the refrigerator until you're ready to use it.

Slow Cooker Balsamic Chicken & Sausage

Ingredients

- 4 Boneless, Skinless Chicken Breasts
- 1 White Onion, Thinly Sliced
- 6 Italian Sausage Links
- Extra Virgin Olive Oil
- 6 Cloves Of Garlic, Chopped
- 1 Tsp. Italian Seasoning
- 1 Tsp. Kosher Salt
- 1 Tsp. Garlic Powder
- 29 Oz. Can Diced Tomatoes
- 15 Oz. Canned Tomato Sauce
- 1 C. Chicken Stock
- ½ C. Balsamic Vinegar

- 1 Tsp. Italian Seasoning
- ½ Tsp. Garlic Powder
- ½ Tsp. Kosher Salt

Directions

1. Lay the chicken in the bottom of your slow cooker and drizzle it with a few tablespoons of olive oil.
2. Add the first set of seasonings directly on the chicken. Don't mix it; just leave it on the top. During the process, it will season the chicken.
3. Put the whole sausage links over the chicken.
4. Layer the sliced onion and the garlic on next.
5. Pour the tomato sauce, tomatoes, stock, and the vinegar into the pot.
6. Top with the second set of seasonings and don't mix it up.
7. Cover and set the slow cook on high for five hours.

Crock Pot Carnitas

Ingredients

- 5 Lb. Pork Loin Roast
- 1 Tsp Garlic Powder
- 1 Tsp Ground Cumin
- 1 Tsp Chili Powder
- 1 Tsp Kosher Salt
- 1 Lime
- 2 Oranges

- 2 C. Chicken Stock
- 1 Tbsp. Adobo
- 2 Tbsp. Tomato Paste
- 4 Garlic Cloves, Crushed
- Butter

Directions

1. Slice the roast into two-inch steaks and leave all the fat in place.
2. Blend together the spices in a large bowl and then toss in the steak pieces a few at a time and coat them in the spices.
3. Heat a skillet or a large pan on medium high and add some butter.
4. Work in batches to ensure it's a quick sear. Add two to three steaks, depending on their size and sear both sides.
5. Move the browned pork to your slow cooker and repeat until all the pieces are done.
6. Once the last batch is seared, bring the stock, adobo, tomato paste, and the garlic cloves together in the pan. Use this to deglaze the pan.
7. Let the seasoned broth simmer a few minutes in the skillet.
8. While the broth is simmering, juice the oranges and the lime and set it aside.
9. After a few minutes of simmering, pour the broth into the slow cooker and add the citrus juices.
10. Cover and set it on low for five hours.
11. If your slow cooker turns off after the timer goes off, let it rest for half an hour. If you have the keep warm setting, then you need to get to the pork immediately, or it will dry out.

12. Shred the meat with some forks or a pastry cutter. Caramelize the shredded meat in order to get the browned edges. Put some shredded meat into a skillet with a little fat and brown or put the meat under a broiler for a few minutes.
13. Then assembled the carnitas and enjoy!

Savory Cinnamon Slow Cooker Chicken

Ingredients

- 2 Lbs. Chicken Breasts
- 2 Bell Peppers Sliced
- 2 Tsp. Paprika
- 1 Onion, Diced
- 4 Cloves Garlic, Minced
- 2 Tsp. Cinnamon
- 1 C. Chicken Broth
- ¼ Tsp. Nutmeg

Directions

1. Combine everything in a gallon freezer bag and make sure the air is out before you seal it.
2. Remove the meal from the freezer the night before you want to cook it and defrost it in the refrigerator.
3. Pour the bag contents into the slow cooker and cook on low for six hours or high for four.
4. Serve.

Greek Stuffed Chicken Breasts

Ingredients

- 6 Boneless Chicken Breasts
- 1 Tbsp. Olive Oil
- ½ Onion, Diced
- ½ Red Pepper, Sliced
- 2 Pepperoncini Peppers, Sliced
- 2 Tsp. Minced Garlic
- 6 Oz. Spinach
- 1 ½ Tsp. Fresh Oregano
- Salt And Pepper
- 1 C. Chicken Stock
- Squeeze Of Lemon
- ½ C. White Wine
- ⅓ C. Feta Cheese

Directions

1. Cut a slit into the center of one side of the chicken breasts so that you make a deep pocket. Generously season them with salt and pepper on either side and set them aside.

2. In a skillet over medium heat, add the oil. Sauté the peppers and the onion for a minute or two or until they begin to sweat. Add the spinach and garlic and cook until the spinach has wilted. Add the fresh oregano and a bit of salt and pepper. Remove it from the heat.

3. If you're using the feta, the stuff a teaspoon into the pocket of the chicken, making sure to put it as far back as you can go. Then spoon in equal amounts of the pepper and spinach mix into the chicken breasts. Add the stuffed breasts to the slow cooker and squeeze a fresh splash of lemon juice over them. Add the stock and wine to the slow cooker. Cover and cook on low for six to eight hours or high for four hours. Top with optional toppings if you'd like, and then enjoy.

Easy Shredded Pork over Caramelized Plantains

- 2 Lbs. Pork Loin
- 1 Onion, Sliced
- 3 C. Beef Broth
- 1 Tsp. Onion Powder
- 1 Tbsp. Garlic Powder
- Salt And Pepper, To Taste
- 4 Brown Plantains, Peeled, Halved The Long Direction
- 1 Tsp. Cinnamon
- 2 Tbsp. Coconut Oil
- Pinch Of Salt
- Pinch Of Allspice
- 4 Tbsp. Canned Coconut Milk

1. Add the pork, onion, beef broth, onion powder, garlic powder, salt, and the pepper to the slow cooker and stir. Cook on low for eight to ten hours. Once the pork is done, use two forks to shred it into pieces.
2. Put a skillet over medium heat and add the coconut oil. Once it's melted and the skillet is hot, add the plantains.
3. Sprinkle with the allspice, cinnamon, and the salt. Cook on either side for four to five minutes or until they're soft.
4. Add them to a food processor and puree them. While the food processor is running, pour in the coconut milk until you have a smooth puree. Taste for seasonings.
5. To serve, add a scoop of the mash to the plates and top with the pork. Garnish with some avocado slices and a littleminced cilantro, if you like.

Coffee Braised Chile Beef

Ingredients

- 1 Beef Roast
- 4 Garlic Cloves, Minced
- 2 Tsp. Cocoa Powder
- 3 Tbsp. Ancho Chile Powder
- 1 Tsp. Oregano
- 1 Tsp. Cumin
- ⅛ Tsp. Cinnamon

- ½ Tsp. Salt, Or To Taste
- ½ Tsp. Chipotle Powder
- ¾ C. Strong Brewed Coffee
- 1 Tbsp. Balsamic Vinegar
- ½ Onion, Thickly Sliced

Directions

1. Combine the ingredients but the beef, onion, coffee, and vinegar in a bowl. Add enough water to it to make a loose paste. Rub the spice mix all over the beef on all sides.
2. Spread the onion on the bottom of the slow cooker. Put the beef over the top and stir the vinegar into the coffee. Pour the coffee mix over the roast.
3. Cook for six to eight hours on low or until it's tender.

Slow Cooker Kimchi Chicken

Ingredients

- 1 C. Low-Sodium Chicken Broth
- 6 Garlic Cloves, Minced
- 4 Scallions, Sliced
- 1 Tbsp. Soy Sauce
- 1 Tbsp. Dark Sesame Oil
- 2 Tsp. Palm Sugar
- 1 Tsp. Ginger, Minced
- 2 Lbs. Boneless Skinless Chicken Thighs
- 2 C. Cabbage Kimchi, Drained

1. Combine all the ingredients but the chicken, scallion greens, and the kimchi in the slow cooker.

2. Put the thighs into the sauce and spoon some over the top of them.

3. Cover and cook them for four to six hours on low.

4. When they're ready to serve, turn the heat up to high and add the kimchi. Cook another twenty minutes and serve garnished with the scallion greens.

Crock Pot Beef Tongue with Roasted Pepper Sauce

Ingredients

- 1 Beef Tongue
- 3 Garlic Cloves, Crushed
- 1 Onion, Sliced
- 3 Bay Leaves
- Water
- Sea Salt And Pepper
- 1 Roasted Serrano Chili Pepper, Diced
- 1 Roasted Red Pepper, Peeled And Diced
- 1 Onion, Diced
- 20 Oz. Tomatoes, Sliced
- 3 Garlic Cloves, Minced
- 6 Oz. Tomato Paste
- 1 Tsp. Oregano

- 1 Tsp. Thyme
- Salt And Pepper To Taste

1. For the tongue, wash the beef under cold water and pat it dry.
2. Line the bottom of the slow cooker with the garlic, onion, and the bay leaves.
3. Put the tongue on the top and generously season it with salt and pepper.
4. Add as much water as necessary to completely submerge it in water.
5. Cover and cook on low for eight hours.
6. Remove it from the slow cooker and remove the skin of the tongue.
7. Shred the beef and serve it with the following sauce recipe.
8. In a saucepan over medium heat, sauté the garlic, onions, red pepper, and the Chile until the onions are clear.
9. Add the rest of the ingredients and stir.
10. Reduce the heat to low and simmer for half an hour.
11. Leave the sauce chunky or put it in a food processor to make a smooth sauce.
12. Serve over the shredded beef and enjoy.

Pork Chop Suey

- 2 Lbs. Pork Stew Meat

- 4 Stalks Of Celery, Sliced
- 1 Onion, Chopped
- 1 Can Of Bamboo Shoots
- 1 Can Of Mushrooms
- ½ C. Of Chicken Stock
- 2 C. Of Snow Peas
- 2 C. Of Green Cabbage
- ½ Package Of Sweet Potato Noodles
- ¼ C. Of Coconut Aminos
- 3 Tbsp. Of Arrowroot Powder
- ½ C. Of Stew Liquid

Directions

1. Heat the oil in a pan and sear the pork on all the sides. Add the celery and onions and mix it all together. Let it cook a few minutes.
2. Put the mix into the slow cooker and add the bamboo shoots, mushrooms, and the chicken stock. Cook on low for seven hours.
3. When the slow cooker is twenty minutes from being done, stem the peas and the cabbage.
4. Boil the noodles for six minutes.
5. Take half a cup of the stew liquid and put it into another pot. Stir in the snow peas, cabbage, and the sweet potato noodles.
6. To make the sauce, combine the stew liquid with the coconut aminos in a saucepot. Whisk in the arrowroot powder and bring it all to a boil. Turn it down to a simmer for three minutes.
7. Pour the sauce on the plates and enjoy.

Chapter Three – Clean Eating, Vegetarian Slow Cooker Dinner Recipes

Springtime Crockpot Minestrone

Ingredients

- 1 Onion, Diced
- 3 Carrots, Peeled And Sliced
- 3 Garlic Cloves, Minced
- 28 Oz. Of Diced Tomatoes
- 30 Oz. Of Cannellini Beans
- 3 C. Low-Sodium Vegetable Stock
- 3 C. Water
- 8 Oz. Of Uncooked Ditalini Pasta
- 12 Asparagus Spears, Cut Into Thirds
- 1 C. Of Frozen Sweet Peas
- 6 Oz. Of Fresh Spinach
- ⅓ C. Romano Cheese, Grated
- Salt And Pepper To Taste

Directions

1. Add the garlic, onions, carrots, and the entire can of the diced tomatoes, beans, stock, and the water to the slow cooker. Cook on low for four to six hours, stirring once if you can.

2. Around ten to fifteen minutes before you serve, add in the asparagus, peas, spinach, and the pasta. Cook on low another ten to fifteen minutes and then stir in the cheese.

3. Taste and season with some salt and pepper. Serve with cheese on top.

Slow Cooker Smoky Sweet Potato and Chickpea Chili with Lime

Ingredients

- 13.5 oz. can of tomato sauce
- 28 oz. can of diced tomatoes
- 28 oz. adobo peppers in sauce
- 2 tbsp. chili powder
- 1 tsp. salt
- 1 tsp. ground cumin
- ½ c. stock
- 1 sweet potato, peeled and cubed
- 4 cloves garlic, minced
- 2 carrots, peeled and diced
- 2 onions, diced
- 38 oz. canned chickpeas, drained and rinsed
- Juice of half a lime
- Avocado
- Sour cream
- Cilantro leaves

- Tortilla chips

1. In the base of your slow cooker, combine the tomato sauce, tomatoes, cumin, chili powder, peppers, salt, and the stock. Mix it until it's combined well.
2. Add in the rest of the ingredients and combine.
3. Cook on low for eight to ten hours.
4. Before you serve, stir in the lime juice gently.
5. Serve with the cilantro, avocado, sour cream, and the chips.

Slow Cooker Black Bean Pumpkin Chili

- 2 14.5 Oz. Cans Plain Diced Tomatoes
- 3 15 Oz. Cans Black Beans, Drained
- 1 C. Pureed Pumpkin
- 2 C. Diced Yellow Onion
- 1 Yellow Bell Pepper, Diced
- 1 Tbsp. Chili Powder
- 1 Tsp. Cumin
- 1 Tsp. Cinnamon
- ¼ Tsp. Nutmeg
- ½ Tsp. Kosher Salt
- ⅛ Tsp. Ground Cloves
- ½ Tsp. Ground Black Pepper

- Cherry Tomatoes
- Avocado
- Cilantro

1. Add everything to a four-quart slow cooker and stir.
2. Cook on low eight to ten hours.
3. Serve with your chosen toppings.

Crock-Pot mushroom stroganoff

- 1 ½ Lbs. Mushrooms, Diced
- 1 Onion, Halved And Sliced
- 3 Cloves Garlic, Minced
- 1 C. Vegetable Stock
- 1 Tbsp. Sour Cream
- 2 Tsp. Smoked Paprika
- Salt And Pepper
- 4 Tbsp. Parsley, Chopped

1. Add the first five ingredients to your slow cooker and mix it well. Cook on high for four hours.
2. After four hours, stir in the sour cream and season it to taste. Serve topped with parsley.

Crockpot Cauliflower Bolognese with Zucchini Noodles

Ingredients

- 1 Head Of Cauliflower, Chopped
- ¾ C. Red Onion, Diced
- 2 Small Garlic Cloves, Minced
- 1 Tsp. Dried Basil Flakes
- 2 Tsp. Dried Oregano Flakes
- 28 Oz. Cans Diced Tomatoes
- ½ C. Vegetable Broth
- Salt And Pepper, To Taste
- ¼ Tsp. Red Pepper Flakes
- 5 Large Zucchinis, Spiralized

Directions

1. Put everything for the Bolognese into a slow cooker. Leave out the zucchini. Put the slow cooker on high and let it cook three and a half hours.
2. When it's done, smash the cauliflower with a potato masher until the florets break up.
3. Spoon the Bolognese over the noodles and serve.

Slow Cooker Creamy Tomato Basil Tortellini Soup

- 1 ¾ C. Diced Carrots
- 1 ¾ C. Diced Yellow Onion
- 5 Cloves Garlic, Minced
- 2 Tbsp. Olive Oil
- 84 oz. canned Whole Roma Tomatoes
- ⅓ C. Chopped Fresh Basil
- 32 Oz. Carton Vegetable Broth
- 2 Bay Leaves
- 1 Tbsp. Granulated Sugar
- Salt And Pepper
- ¾ C. Heavy Cream
- 16 Oz. Refrigerated Three Cheese Tortellini
- Parmesan, Shredded

1. Heat the oil in a skillet over medium heat and sauté the onion and carrots for three to four minutes. Add the garlic and sauté another minute. Pour the mix into a six or seven-quart slow cooker with the broth, tomatoes, bay leaves, basil, and the sugar. Stir and season to taste with salt and pepper. Cover and cook on low six to seven hours or in on high three hours.

2. Remove the bay and puree the mix well in a blender. Stir in the tortellini and cook on high for fifteen more minutes. Reduce the

heat to warm and stir in the cream. Serve topped with the cheese and some fresh basil.

Slow Cooker Vegan White Bean Stew

Ingredients

- 2 Lbs. White Beans
- 3 Celery Stalks, Diced
- 2 Carrots, Peeled And Diced
- 1 Onion, Diced
- 3 Cloves Garlic, Minced Or Chopped
- 1 Tsp. Dried Rosemary
- 1 Tsp. Thyme
- 1 Tsp. Oregano
- 1 Bay Leaf
- 12 C. Water
- 2 Tbsp. Salt
- Pepper
- 28 Oz. Diced Tomatoes
- 6 C. Roughly Chopped Spinach
- Rice, For Serving

Directions

1. Sort through and rinse the beans a few times in cold water. Add them to the slow cooker with the celery, diced carrots, onions, dried herbs, and the bay leaf. Add the water. Cover and cook on high three to four hours or on low for eight to ten hours. Remove

the lid and add the salt and pepper and the tomatoes. Let it cook for another hour and a half or until the beans have softened.

2. Stir in the chopped spinach before serving.

3. Serve it hot over rice.

Quinoa Black Bean Crockpot Stuffed Peppers

Ingredients

- 6 Bell Peppers
- 1 C. Uncooked Quinoa, Rinsed
- 14 Oz. Can Black Beans, Rinsed And Drained
- 14 Oz. Can Refried Beans
- 1½ C. Red Enchilada Sauce
- 1 Tsp. Cumin
- 1 Tsp. Onion Powder
- 1 Tsp. Chili Powder
- ½ Tsp. Garlic Salt
- 1½ C. Pepper Jack Cheese, Shredded
- Avocado
- Cilantro
- Sour Cream

Directions

1. Cut the tops off the peppers and scrape out the seeds and the ribs.

2. In a bowl, combine the beans, quinoa, spices, enchilada sauce, and a cup of the cheese. Fill the peppers with the quinoa mix.

3. Pour half a cup of water into the bottom of your slow cooker. Put the peppers in so they're sitting in the water. Cover and cook on low for six hours or on high for three hours. Remove the lid and distribute the rest of the cheese over the tops of the peppers. Cover again for a few minutes to melt the cheese.

4. Serve topped with the avocado, sour cream, and cilantro.

Slow Cooker Sweet Potato Soup

Ingredients

- 5 C. Low Sodium Vegetable Broth
- 3 Sweet Potatoes, Peeled And Chopped
- 1 C. Chopped Onion
- 2 Cloves Of Garlic, Crushed
- 2 Stalks Of Celery, Chopped
- 1 C. Of Rice Milk
- 1 Tsp. McCormick Pinch Perfect Seasoning
- 1 Tsp. Dried Tarragon
- 2 C. Packed Baby Spinach
- 8 Tbsp. Sliced Almonds
- Salt And Pepper

Directions

1. Add the potatoes, broth, celery, onion, and garlic to a slow cooker.

2. Cook on low for eight hours or high for five hours.

3. Turn it off and add the rice milk, seasoning, and tarragon. Blend for a minute with an immersion blender or until it's smooth.

4. Stir in the spinach, cover, and let it rest for twenty minutes or until the spinach is wilted.

5. Ladle it into soup bowls and top with the sliced almonds, peppers, and salt.

Slow Cooker Enchilada Quinoa

Ingredients

1. 15 Oz. Can Black Beans, Drained And Rinsed

2. 15 Oz. Can Yellow Corn, Drained And Rinsed

3. 30 Oz. Can Of Red Enchilada Sauce, Divided

4. 15 Oz. Can Of Diced Fire Roasted Tomatoes And Green Chiles

5. 1 C. Raw Quinoa

6. ½ C. Water

7. 4 Oz. Cream Cheese

8. Salt And Pepper To Taste

9. 1 C. Mexican Style Cheese, Shredded

10. Diced Tomatoes

11. Chopped Cilantro

12. Sour Cream

13. Diced Avocado

Directions

1. Add the beans, corn, and a can of the sauce, tomatoes, water, quinoa, cream cheese, and salt and pepper to the slow cooker. Stir it together.

2. Pour the rest of the sauce on top and sprinkle it with the shredded cheese. Cover and cook on high for four to five hours or low for five to seven hours.

3. Uncover and top with the remaining ingredient before serving.

Chapter Four – Indian Slow Cooker Recipes

Indian Ground Lamb Curry

Ingredients

- 2 Tbsp. Grass-Fed Ghee
- 1 Lb. Ground Lamb
- 1 C. Peas
- 2 Potatoes, Chopped
- 1 Onion, Diced
- 3 Carrots, Chopped
- 4 Cloves Garlic, Minced
- 1" Fresh Ginger, Minced
- 4 Tomatoes, Chopped
- 2 Serrano Peppers
- 1 Tbsp. Coriander Powder
- 1 Tsp. Paprika
- ½ Tsp. Cumin Powder
- 1 Tsp. Meat Masala
- ½ Tsp. Kashmiri Chili Powder
- ¼ Tsp. Turmeric Powder
- 1 Tsp. Salt
- ½ Tsp. Black Pepper
- 1 C. Tomato Sauce

- Cilantro, For Garnish

1. Melt the ghee in a pan over medium heat and sauté the onions until they're golden brown.
2. Add the garlic, ginger, and the serrano pepper. Stir-fry for a minute and then add the tomatoes. Cover and cook for five minutes.
3. Add the spices and stir-fry them for a minute before adding the ground lamb.
4. Once the meat is completely browned, add it to your slow cooker along with the carrots, peas, potatoes, and the tomato sauce.
5. Cook it on low for four to five hours.

Dum Aloo

Ingredients

- 12 Baby Potatoes
- 1 Onion, Sliced
- 1 Tbsp. Minced Ginger
- 2 Tbsp. Raisins
- 1 Tbsp. Minced Garlic
- 1 Tbsp. Kasoori Methi
- 1 Tsp. Oil
- 4 Green Chilies, Slit
- 1" Cinnamon Stick
- 1 Bay Leaf

- 2 Cloves
- ½ Tsp. Garam Masala
- ¼ Tsp. Turmeric Powder
- ½ Tsp. Chilli Powder
- ¼ Tsp. Asafetida
- ⅓ C. Water
- ½ C. Thick Plain Yogurt
- Salt To Taste
- Cilantro, Chopped

Directions

1. Scrub and peel the potatoes. Prick them with a fork all over. This step is important so that the potatoes absorb the flavors of the curry.

2. Add a teaspoon of the base to the slow cooker and brush it on all the bottom and sides. This prevents the curry from sticking and helps the potatoes obtain a sear. You can spray them with some non-stick cooking spray, too. Add the potatoes in a single layer on the bottom of your slow cooker. Turn it on high and leave it on until you prepare the rest of the ingredients.

3. Slice the ginger, onion, green chilies and the onion. Layer them on the potatoes. Top with the garam masala, cloves, cinnamon, and the bay leaf. Top with the spice powders of garam masala, turmeric powder, chili powder, salt, and the asafetida. Add enough water to reach halfway through the potatoes but not so much it covers them.

4. Close the lid of the slow cooker and cook for eight to ten hours on low.

5. Switch the slow cooker off and remove the lid. Add the kasoori methi, raisins, and the yogurt. Mix it up to combine. The residual heat will cook the yogurt. Sprinkle with the chopped cilantro and serve.

Slow Cooker Indian Potato Kale Soup

Ingredients

- 3 C. Vegetable Broth
- 1 C. Chickpeas
- 4 Tomatoes, Diced
- 1 Lb. Potatoes, Diced
- 1 C. Red Onion, Diced
- 2 Tbsp. Curry Paste
- 1 Tbsp. Minced Garlic
- 2 Tsp. Coriander, Ground
- 1 Tsp. Garam Masala
- ½ Lb. Kale, Chopped
- Salt And Pepper, To Taste

Directions

1. Pour some of the olive oil into the bottom of your slow cooker. Add everything but the kale and the salt and pepper. Stir. Cook it on low for six to eight hours. Chop the kale in the meantime.

2. Use an immersion blender to blend half the soup until it's creamy. Add the chopped kale and cook on high for thirty minutes or until the kale is tender. Season with some salt and pepper and serve.

Indian Butter Chicken

- 4 C. Cubed Chicken
- 1 Tsp. Indian Chili Powder
- 1 Tbsp. Lemon Juice
- ½ Tsp. Salt
- 1 C. Greek Yogurt
- 1 Tsp. Mild Indian Chili Powder
- 2 Tbsp. Garlic Paste
- 2 Tbsp. Ginger Paste
- ½ Tsp. Ground Garam Masala
- 2 Tbsp. Mustard Oil Or Olive Oil
- ½ Tsp. Salt
- 4 Tbsp. Unsalted Butter
- 3 Cardamom Pods
- 6 Peppercorns
- 4 Cloves
- 1" Cinnamon Stick
- 1 Tbsp. Garlic Paste
- 1 Tbsp. Ginger Paste
- 5 Green Chilies, Chopped

- 2 C. Tomato Puree

- 1 Tbsp. Indian Chili Powder

- ½ Tsp. Ground Garam Masala

- 2 Tbsp. Mild Honey

- 1 C. Cayenne Pepper, To Taste

- Chopped Fresh Cilantro, For Garnish

Directions

1. Broil the chicken and put everything in the slow cooker and cook on low for eight hours.

Vegetarian Indian Falafel Recipe

Ingredients

- ½ Onion, Chopped

- 10 Oz. Black-Eyed Peas

- 3 Tbsp. Curry

- 2 Cloves Minced Garlic

- 1 Egg

- 2 Tsp. House Seasoning Blend

- Juice From 1 Lime

- ¾ C. Bread Crumbs

- 2 Tbsp. Olive Oil

1. Put everything but the bread crumbs into your food processor and pulse until it makes a chunky falafel mix. Add the crumbs and pulse until it balls up.

2. Put some olive oil in the bottom of the slow cooker. Ball up ten of the falafel balls and drop them into the slow cooker. Cook on high for two to five hours.

3. They're done when they've turned golden brown. Flip them halfway through to get a more even browning.

4. Serve with some yogurt sauce or tzatziki.

Vegetarian Baked Potato Ball Curry

Ingredients

- 1 Lb. Potatoes, Baked And Mashed
- 2 Tbsp. Red Onions, Finely Chopped
- 1 Tsp. Chili Powder
- ½ Tsp. Turmeric
- 2 Tbsp. Cilantro, Finely Chopped
- ½ Tsp. Salt
- 1 Tsp. Chili Powder
- ¼ Tsp. Cayenne Pepper
- 1 Tsp. Ground Coriander
- ¼ Tsp. Salt
- 1 ¼ C. Water
- 2 Tbsp. Oil
- 2 Onions, Minced

- 6 Cloves Garlic, Minced
- 2 Tbsp. Tomato Paste
- 2 Tbsp. Yogurt
- ¼ C. Cilantro, Chopped

Directions

1. Preheat your oven to 375 degrees.
2. Grease a baking sheet.
3. In a bowl, mix the first six ingredients together.
4. Roll the mix into one inch balls and space them evenly apart on the baking sheet.
5. Bake for twenty minutes or until they're brown and crispy. Set them aside.
6. Combine the remaining ingredients in a slow cooker. Put the koftas on top of the sauce in the slow cooker and cook on low for eight hours.

Slow Cooker Lamb Curry

Ingredients

- C. Cubed Lamb
- 1 Onion, Chopped
- 4 Oz. Mushrooms, Chopped
- 2 Tbsp. Curry
- 2 Cloves Garlic, Minced
- 2 Tbsp. Coconut Oil
- 2 Tbsp. Olive Oil

- 1 Tbsp. Garam Masala
- 1 Tsp. Ginger
- 1 Tsp. Salt
- 1 Tbsp. Oregano
- 2 Large Baking Potatoes, Cubed
- Oz. Tomato Paste
- 1 C. Coconut Milk
- 1 Bunch Cilantro, Chopped
- Brown Rice, Cooked

Directions

1. Put all the ingredients, except the coconut milk and cilantro, into the slow cooker and cook on low five to seven hours. Stir in the milk and serve it over rice, garnished with the cilantro.

Masaman Curry

Ingredients

- 8 Oz. Seitan
- ½ C. Vegetable Broth
- ½ C. Coconut Milk
- 1 Tbsp. Masaman Curry Paste
- ¾ Tsp. Salt
- 1 Tbsp. Sugar
- 1 C. Onion, Chopped
- 1 C. Potato, Cubed
- Cardamon Pods

- 1 Cinnamon Stick
- 2 Bay Leaves
- ¼ C. Cashews For Garnish
- Cilantro, For Garnish

Directions

1. Pour some of the oil into the bottom of the slow cooker. Put the broth and seitan in the bottom of the slow cooker. Mix the milk and curry paste together in a bowl. Mix in the sugar and the salt. Put the chopped potato and onion in the slow cooker. Wrap the rest of the spices in a cheesecloth and put them in the slow cooker.

2. Pour the coconut milk mix over the seitan and the vegetables. Cook it on low for five to eight hours, adding more broth if you need to. Stir it once halfway through. Serve it over rice with some cilantro and cashews as a garnish.

Slow Cooker Chicken Tikka Masala

Ingredients

- 2 Lbs. Chicken Thighs
- 1 C. Canned Coconut Milk
- 2 C. Crushed Tomatoes
- 1 Tbsp. Ginger Root, Minced
- 3 Cloves Garlic, Minced
- ½ Onion, Thinly Sliced
- 1 Tbsp. Garam Masala

- 1 Tsp. Ground Coriander
- ½ Tsp. Kosher Salt
- 1 Tsp. Ground Cumin
- ¼ Tsp Red Chili Flakes
- 1 Tbsp. Palm Sugar
- 2 Tbsp. Butter
- Coconut Oil
- Cilantro For Garnish

Directions

1. Prepare and clean the chicken thighs, removing the excess skin and fat. Put them in a bowl and coat them with a tablespoon of the garam masala.
2. Heat a pan to high and melt a few tablespoons of coconut oil in it.
3. Sear the thighs, beginning with the skin side down. Sear them on both sides and then put them in the slow cooker.
4. Thinly slice half the onion and lay it on top of the thighs.
5. In the pan, melt two tablespoons of butter with the minced ginger and the garlic over medium heat.
6. When the garlic and the ginger sizzle, add the crushed tomatoes and coconut milk.
7. The spices go in next, along with the palm sugar.
8. Simmer for a few minutes or until the spices are well mixed in, and the sauce starts to bubble.
9. Pour the sauce over the thighs and the onions in the slow cooker.
10. Cover and set the slow cooker on low. Cook for three to four hours.

Kheer in Slow Cooker

Ingredients

- 8 C. Milk
- ½ C. Uncooked Rice
- Tbsp. Sugar
- ¼ C. Slivered Almonds
- ¼ C. Golden Raisins
- ¼ Tsp. Cardamom Powder

Directions

1. Rinse the rice.
2. Put everything in the slow cooker and set it to high. Stir it after an hour and make sure the rice isn't clumping together.
3. Cook for two more hours, stir again and cook another two hours on high or low for four hours.
4. The longer you cook it, the creamier it will become.
5. Turn the slow cooker off and allow it to cool. Refrigerate it and serve it chilled or warm with a little nutmeg on top of it.

Chapter Five - Crock Pot Dump Meals

Slow Cooker Root Vegetable Stew

Ingredients

- 1 White Onion, Chopped
- 1 Lb. Butternut Squash, Chopped
- 1 Lb. Parsnips, Chopped
- 1 Lb. Carrots, Chopped
- 1 Lb. Sweet Potatoes, Chopped
- 2 Celery Ribs, Stems Removed And Chopped
- 1 Lb. Yukon Gold Potatoes, Chopped
- Cloves Garlic, Sliced
- 3 C. Chicken Or Vegetable Broth
- 1 Bay Leaf
- 1 Tbsp. Fresh Sage Leaves, Minced
- 1 Tsp. Black Pepper
- ½ Tsp. Sea Salt
- 2 C. Chopped Fresh Kale

Directions

1. Add everything but the kale to the slow cooker and cook on low for six to eight hours.
2. Remove the bay leaf and stir in the kale. Let it cook another ten minutes or until the kale has wilted. Season to taste.

3. Turn off the slow cooker and serve immediately.

Slow Cooker Sweet Fire Chicken

Ingredients

- Boneless Skinless Chicken Breasts, Diced
- 1 Can Pineapple Chunks, Drained
- 1 Red Bell Pepper, Chopped
- 2 Tsp. Minced Garlic
- ⅔ C. Sugar
- 2 Tsp. Crushed Red Pepper Flakes
- 1 C. Water
- 2 Tbsp. Sweet Red Chili Sauce
- ½ Tsp. Salt
- 4 Tbsp. Cold Water
- 3 Tbsp. Corn Starch

Directions

1. Add the red peppers, chicken, and the pineapple to a greased slow cooker.

2. In a bowl, whisk the remaining ingredients but the cold water and the cornstarch together. Pour the sauce into the slow cooker and stir it well. Cover it and cook it on high for two to three hours or low for four to five hours.

3. Around half an hour before it's done, take the lid off the slow cooker. Whisk the cornstarch and water together and slowly stir it

into the slow cooker. Cover and cook another half an hour or until you're ready to serve.

4. Serve it with some steamed rice, if you like.

BBQ Pork Ribs

- 3 Lbs. Boneless Pork Ribs
- ½ Onion, Thinly Sliced
- 3 Cloves Garlic, Minced
- ¼ C. Brown Sugar
- 1½ C. Barbecue Sauce
- ½ C. Apple Sauce
- Salt And Pepper

1. Lightly salt and pepper the pork ribs on both sides. Add everything to the slow cooker. Gently mix it and cook on low for five to six hours. Remove it from the slow cooker and discard the juices. Top with half a cup of the barbecue sauce. Serve.

2. To freeze, salt and pepper the ribs. Mix everything else together and add it all to a freezer safe bag. Label and freeze. To cook it, thaw the bag and then add it to the slow cooker as directed.

Lemon Garlic Dump Chicken

Ingredients

- 2 Tsp. Minced Garlic
- ¼ C. Olive Oil
- 1 Tbsp. Parsley Flakes
- 2 Tbsp. Lemon Juice
- Chicken Breasts

Directions

1. Put all the ingredients into a one-gallon bag. Put all the ingredients into the bag.
2. After you seal, turn it around a few times to distribute everything. Freeze it flat.
3. To cook it, put everything but the bag into the slow cooker and cook on low for six to eight hours or high for four to six hours.

Slow Cooker Honey Sesame Chicken

Ingredients

- 2 Cloves Garlic, Minced
- 1 Onion, Diced
- ½ C. Honey
- ½ C. Soy Sauce
- ¼ C. Ketchup
- 2 Tbsp. Vegetable Oil
- ¼ Tsp. Crushed Red Pepper Flakes

- 2 Lbs. Boneless, Skinless Chicken Thighs
- Salt And Pepper, To Taste
- 1 Green Onion, Sliced
- Sesame Seeds, For Garnish

Directions

1. In a bowl, combine the garlic, onion, soy sauce, honey, vegetable oil, ketchup, and the red pepper.

2. Season the thighs with some salt and pepper to taste. Put the thighs into the slow cooker and add the sauce over the top. Toss to combine and cover. Cook on low for heat three hours and thirty minutes.

3. Remove the thighs from the slow cooker and shred them before returning them to the pot with the juices. Cover and keep warm another half an hour.

4. Serve immediately garnished with sesame seeds and green onions.

Slow Cooker Broccoli Beef

Ingredients

- 1 ½ Lbs. Flank Steak, Chopped
- 1 C. Beef Broth
- ⅔ C. Soy Sauce
- ⅓ C. Brown Sugar
- 1 Tbsp. Sesame Oil
- 1 Tbsp. Minced Garlic

- ¼ Tsp. Red Chili
- C. Broccoli Florets
- 2 Tbsp. Corn Starch
- 4 Tbsp. Cold Water

Directions

1. Grease the inside of your slow cooker and add the beef broth, steak, soy sauce, sesame oil, brown sugar, chili flakes, and garlic. Cover and cook on high for two to three hours or on low for four to five hours.

2. Just before serving, uncover the slow cooker. Whisk the cornstarch and water together in a bowl and dissolve it. Add it to the slow cooker and stir. Cover and let it cook another twenty minutes.

3. Just before you serve, put the broccoli into a microwave safe bowl and fill it with half an inch of water. Put it in the microwave for three minutes. Drain and stir it into the slow cooker.

Slow Cooker Black Bean Soup

Ingredients

- 3 C. Dried Black Beans, Soaked
- 1 Tbsp. Olive Oil
- 1 Yellow Onion, Chopped
- Garlic Cloves, Minced
- 1 Red Bell Pepper, Chopped
- 1 Tbsp. Salt

- ½ C. Chopped Cilantro
- 8 C. Water

1. In a skillet over medium heat, add the olive oil. Add the onion and the red pepper and sauté for four to five minutes. Add the garlic and sauté another minute or until it's fragrant.
2. Pour the beans into the slow cooker, and then add the onion and pepper mix. Add the cilantro, water, and the salt. Stir to combine. Cook in the slow cooker for eight hours on low or four hours on high.
3. Serve it warm with fresh cilantro, rice, sour cream, cheese, tomatoes, salsa, or avocado.

White Chicken Chili

- C. Chicken Broth
- 4 C. Cooked Shredded Chicken
- 28 Oz. Canned Great Northern Beans, Drained
- 2 C. Salsa Verde
- 2 Tsp. Ground Cumin
- Diced Avocado
- Shredded Cheese
- Chopped Fresh Cilantro
- Chopped Green Onions
- Crumbled Tortilla Chips

- Sour Cream

1. Add the chicken broth, two breasts, salsa, beans, and the cumin to the slow cooker. Stir to combine. Cook on low for six to eight hours or on high for three to four hours.
2. Shred the chicken.
3. Serve warm with your desired toppings.

Slow Cooker Potato and Corn Chowder

- 24 Oz. Red Potato, Diced
- 16 Oz. Package Frozen Corn
- 3 Tbsp. All-Purpose Flour
- C. Chicken Stock
- 1 Tsp. Dried Thyme
- 1 Tsp. Dried Oregano
- ½ Tsp. Garlic Powder
- ½ Tsp. Onion Powder
- Salt And Pepper
- 2 Tbsp. Unsalted Butter
- ¼ C. Heavy Cream

1. Put the potatoes and the corn into the slow cooker and stir in the flour. Gently toss it to combine. Stir in the thyme, stock, oregano, onion powder, garlic powder, and the salt and pepper.
2. Cover and cook on low for seven to eight hours or high for three to four hours. Stir in the heavy cream and butter when it's done.
3. Serve.

Honey Soy Pork Tenderloin Recipe

- ¼ C. Olive Oil
- 1 C. Chicken Stock Or Broth
- ¼ C. Soy Sauce
- ½ C. Honey
- 3 Tbsp. Steak Seasoning
- 2 Cloves Minced Garlic
- Pinch Ground Ginger
- Pinch Red Pepper Flakes
- 3 Lbs. Pork Tenderloin

1. Spray your slow cooker with some nonstick cooking spray.
2. Mix the chicken broth, oil, soy sauce, steak seasoning, honey, ginger, garlic, and the red pepper flake sin a bowl.

3. Add the pork tenderloin to the slow cooker and pour the oil mixture over the pork tenderloin. Set the slow cook for six hours on low.

Conclusion

Once you're done making your delicious meal, don't forget to wash out the slow cooker for tomorrow's breakfast, lunch, or dinner! Make sure to never use anything abrasive to clean your slow cooker insert because you can scratch and damage it. If you find something has burnt to the bottom of the slow cooker, simply put water in it and let it cook on low overnight. In the morning, the burnt remnants will wash right out!

I hope you enjoyed the recipes you found in this book!

If you did, please leave a review at your online eBook retailer's website.

Thank you for reading!